The Disturbing Truth: Inside Pioneer Manor

TAMMY RECTOR

TAMMY RECTOR

FOREWORD

I was harassed in the workplace, at Pioneer Manor, over a period of two years. During that time, not one person stood up for me or intervened. Everyone turned a blind eye, while I was driven into depression, and ultimately poverty.

The City of Greater Sudbury failed me, as did WSIB, the Greater Sudbury Police, and the Canadian Union of Public Employees. Pioneer Manor failed to acknowledge the harassment and bullying in the workplace, which they claim they have a zero tolerance policy for.

Let me start with this: I have dedicated my life to helping people.

When I made the decision to become a Personal Support Worker, I knew with great certainty that I couldn't find a more suitable career for someone with a heart as big as mine.

I am compassionate. I am motivated. I possess the drive and inspiration to make a difference in the world. I was also born with only one hand, but that didn't deter me from fulfilling my dream.

The entire forty-six years I've been alive, I have dedicated to helping people. Eight of those years were spent at Pioneer Manor, in Sudbury, Ontario—a nursing home whose vision is to "offer residents dignity, respect and care that promotes their comfort and quality of life". The largest facility of its kind in Northern Ontario, whose core values include a promise to "value the residents' rights, as defined in the Long-Term Care Homes Act."

Except they don't. Nor do they value their employees' rights as defined in the Ontario Human Rights Code.

Prior to working at Pioneer Manor, I was employed without any problems, at various other long term health care facilities. I have maintained the highest level of professionalism and I have a proven track record of doing what is asked of me, and more.

When I originally started working for the company in 2006, Pioneer Manor was an acceptable place to work, from what I could tell. During my employment at Pioneer Manor I worked hard, showing up on time, putting my whole heart into my work. I was an excellent employee and had a clean record to prove it. I helped out when I could—if I finished my work before others, I helped them with their residents, as well—and I was never limited by the use of only one hand. I rarely called in sick, and if I did, it was for good reason. I went above and beyond any chance I was given, and always gave 150%, though my efforts went unnoticed—which was fine by me, because I wasn't doing it for any type of recognition—I put my whole heart into my career for the 433 residents of this long-term care facility.

I was proud to represent Pioneer Manor and hoped to retire there. Everything changed on a Sunday morning in March of 2011.

Like everyone else in the world, I, too, enjoy a Sunday morning coffee and a relaxing day off. However, if the well-being of 433 residents was in question due to lack of staff, I was most certainly ready to give up my relaxing day off, as I had done many times in the past. In fact, one of my supervisors named Jane admitted that she always called me first instead of following the call in protocol, simply because she knew I would say yes and she didn't want to waste time calling others who would likely say no.

My phone rang early on this particular Sunday morning in March of 2011—it was the supervisor on shift, asking if I could come in to cover for someone who had called in sick for their shift an area called Killarney. I accepted, as the supervisor probably knew I would—I had hardly ever turned down a shift. I set my coffee aside, got dressed, and headed into work for this shift that I hadn't been originally scheduled for. Another effort that would likely go unnoticed.

I started my shift in Killarney as directed. There was also a shortage of staff in The Lodge, which is the Alzheimer's unit. Six employees had already been asked to fill in for that area. Those six employees had already said no. One of those employees was a woman named Phalyn Sproule, who had the least seniority out of the six employees, and knowing she could be forced to, she made it clear that if she had to work in The Lodge she would leave.

It is very well-known that no one wants to work in The Lodge because several of the employees in there are *bullies*. They have written warning after written warning on each of their employee files for this reason.

Then they heard that I was in the building. Now, forty-five minutes into my shift, Amada, who was the supervisor on shift, asked me to work in The Lodge. I accepted—and to this day, I realize that was a mistake, because that is when everything started.

Please, let me reiterate; this weekend incident occurred in 2011. I had been employed with Pioneer Manor since 2006 and I had never had a problem with anyone at work before this. I always went in on time, worked my shift, and went home. I even met a few people at Pioneer Manor whom I would have considered friends back then.

As I walked into The Lodge, I encountered Michelle O'Connell. She immediately looked at Krista Saile and said, "Oh, you can have her."

Unsure of what that even meant, I brushed it off and said "let me know what you want me to do."

The morning progressed.

The breakfast feeding for residents was significantly behind schedule, and a resident had taken a fall, both due to the lack of staff in the area, but a rumor quickly spread that accused me of being the reason residents had not been fed, even though I had already worked forty-five minutes of my shift in a different department. I was not late for my shift, as implied by the circulating fabrication. I had been called in on what was supposed to be my Sunday off, and I still made it on time for the start of the shift. I had worked for forty-five minutes in the department that I was asked to cover for, and then I had been moved to The Lodge.

I was not late for work, and the fact that breakfast was behind was absolutely not my fault.

The morning continued. Krista was supposed to stay in the dining room so that I could help Antonella Alfarano, but she was nowhere to be found. I was caring for a resident during the resident's morning feed, Antonella became visibly upset that I wasn't able to help her even though she was well aware I could not let the resident eat alone, for safety reasons and due to policy.

I was also told to provide care to the last four residents at the same time, including a resident who specifically required two personal support workers;

something that happened quite regularly at Pioneer Manor.

As per policy, I stayed with the resident I was helping.

Krista Saile and Michelle O'Connell were very slow getting their work done. In a fast paced environment like long-term health care, it is imperative that everyone pull their own weight to avoid delay and make sure all residents receive proper care, but on this particular morning, neither Krista nor Michelle were pulling their own.

In my opinion, Krista Saile smelled of alcohol on her breath, and I found it was apparent that the other workers in this department were hung-over.

It was heavily implied that I should be picking up more of the work—when, still, I had to continue with my client. I said no. I explained that I would finish up with my resident and then continue to help as much as I could with the other residents.

Michelle told me flat out that I needed to pick up the rest of the workload because I apparently *did nothing all morning.* Her tone was intimidating and threatening. Both her tone and actions were witnessed by Sarah Brown and Antonella Alfarano who were also present, and followed Michelle's lead as she bullied me—they did not stand up for me. I believe they were afraid that Michelle and Krista would target them next if they said anything to defend me.

I told other employees in the area that I was going to speak with a supervisor because of this comment and the insinuation that I should have been doing all the work on my own. I approached Amanda, the Registered Nurse and Supervisor who was in charge and asked her what she wanted me to do.

When I returned, Krista and Michelle had collaborated in fabricating a story, both saying that I had become irate, thrown a chair and slammed doors in a fit of rage. Nothing could have been further from the truth—there aren't even any doors in this area that can be slammed.

Feeling defeated, I confronted Krista Saile and Michelle O'Connell about this in front of Amanda, and Krista admitted to her that I had done nothing wrong and

Michelle stood laughing the whole time, and texting on her phone.

The day went on as normal afterwards and I was able to finish my shift without any other incident.

* * *

I returned to work on Monday for my regular shift. During this shift, the girls from The Lodge approached the coordinator, Angela Phillips, and told her they would not work with me because of my poor attitude and lack of team effort.

Shortly into my shift on Monday, I encountered Angela Phillips, the Program Coordinator, in the hallway and decided to voice my opinion about how I felt, and that

I had been accused of being late, not pulling my weight, and throwing a chair.

"I would like to speak with you about what happened this weekend," I said.

Angela immediately threw her hand up in my face and said, "Speak to me after your meeting I booked for you with Glenda and make sure you have a Union Rep with you." She had clearly heard what had happened, and refused to hear what I had to say about the events that took place.

Glenda Gauthier is the Manager of Resident Care and I was surprised when two weeks went by and I still hadn't heard from her. I finally called her on the phone and asked her to come meet with me at the office to speak about the initial incident at the Lodge. I thought she should have taken the situation more seriously.

In the meantime, the two bullies in question, Michelle O'Connell (née Mallette) and Krista Saile, cursed at me, giggled at me to intimidate me, and made it quite obvious that they were speaking about me behind my back, by speaking loudly and making sure I overheard my name being said.

They came over to the area where I was working, solely to make me feel uncomfortable and threatened. They had cornered me in the building on two separate occasions—to tell me that I'd better *keep my mouth shut,* and another time just stare at me, purely to intimidate me.

On one occasion, witnessed by several day staff as well, I was punching out that the morning and they were both standing by the punch clock, where there were cameras. Michelle shouted loudly, "You're not going to get away with this, bitch. You're going to get fired." Kristina Fink, who became my Disability Manager, claimed the cameras didn't show anything but she did admit that Michelle punched in at 6:54am, then I punched in at 6:55am, and Krista followed, also at 6:55am—which proved that all three of us were there at the same time.

This behavior continued regularly and intimidated me to such a degree that I forgot the code to punch out on several occasions.

It was very much a "fight or flight" feeling for me. I felt attacked on so many occasions and feared for my own safety.

While all of this is going on, I continued to work my shifts as an exemplary Personal Support Worker, and then I would sit in my vehicle for half an hour to forty-five minutes, crying and upset, before I could drive myself back home.

* * *

While waiting for the initial meeting with Glenda Gauthier and following the advice of a medical doctor in the Emergency Department at the hospital, I was put on modified duty on May 19, 2011, because I had been injured—hit in the head by a client, sustaining a concussion.

When I finally went to Glenda on June 10, 2011, Glenda informed me that she had not even been made aware that anything was going on or that she was supposed to have a meeting with me so either Angela never informed Glenda as should have, or Glenda was lying to my face.

Glenda agreed to have a meeting with me and I accepted graciously, but then it took a long two weeks before I was given the opportunity to finally meet with Glenda.

I was working my shift, and I was randomly pulled into Angela Phillips' office, with Glenda Gauthier, two whole weeks after the initial Sunday incident. Two entire weeks, where Michelle and Krista were able to continue to harass me; pointing, laughing, intimidating. At this time, I was told I did not require union representation, and off the record, Glenda and Angela both explained that they were aware of the bullying that went on, instigated by Michelle O'Connell (née Mallette). They informed me that they would *get Michelle on their own terms*, without my involvement—but then they did nothing, and the harassment continued, escalating quickly.

* * *

After the Sunday in 2011, the harassment continued over an unacceptable period of time.

But I persevered.

At one point, Mike Brady, the Union Manager at CUPE (Canadian Union of Public Employees), took me aside and explained that the girls in The Lodge were being told to bully or they would lose their jobs. Though I never found out for certain who he meant was telling the girls this, in my opinion it was implied that Glenda was encouraging Michelle and Krista to bully everyone else, and possibly others.

During one of the shifts that I was working on modified duty, Glenda began screaming at me in front of both clients and my co-workers. She embarrassed me and made me feel like an idiot—more harassment, in this already toxic environment. This screaming incident was so bad that afterwards Glenda was told to apologize to me by Tony Parmar.

Still, the harassment continued and numerous incidents occurred.

Another notable incident happened during a shift the following year in January 2012, Krista walked over to the front desk where I was working, sat down, stayed for about five minutes without saying a word, then got up and left. She stared at me the entire time. It was obvious that this had been done just to intimidate me, as Krista would have no other reason to be at the front desk.

Michelle did the same thing, several times—often walking up behind me, and sitting so close to me that she was touching my arm. She would sit in silence, not doing anything, with no reason to be there—as a method of intimidation.

The incidents continued.

More giggling.

More cursing.

More intimidation.

More harassment than anyone should have to endure.

And management ignored it, or encouraged it.

* * *

I would like to point out how unorganized Pioneer Manor is, and expose the skeletons that they hide.

At one point, several residents were assigned to me for dinner, but I was assigned to a different dining room. The fact that I was assigned to a different dining room with other clients meant that the staff in the other dining room would have to feed the residents I was assigned to, because as per policy, I could not leave the ones I was with. A woman named Veronica was working in the dining room, which made her responsible to feed them—otherwise they'd go without eating. However, Veronica refused to feed them.

I had to take extra time out to feed them. I reported this mix up to Angela, who said I was lucky I had fed them, otherwise she would have disciplined me— even though policy states it was the responsibility of the available dining room staff, who in this case was Veronica.

In addition to this incident, and certainly more concerning, an employee named Gilles Aubin stole money via cheques from a resident. He was caught when a resident passed away. In his disciplinary meeting, he told Management that I had told him to do it—which was completely untrue. I was called into a meeting with Gilles's Union Representative, Dave. I truthfully explained that I had nothing to do with it. Dave twisted the story when he relayed it back to Gilles, and told Gilles that I had thrown him under the bus—when in fact I had simply told the truth about the situation. Gilles asked Pioneer Manor to lay him off instead of terminating him so that he would not lose his entire career, but the family of the resident insisted that he be fired or they would press charges in order for this to not happen to anyone else.

* * *

On March 5, 2012, I contacted the Sudbury Regional Police regarding the harassment and bullying that was occurring on a regular basis.

Responding to this claim, an officer from the Greater Sudbury Police came out to Pioneer Manor and met with Michelle and Krista to discuss my formal complaint. A meeting was held with both of the employees, the Police Officer, and Angela Phillips. Angela defended the actions of Krista and Michelle to the officer, but the officer said "I will arrest them right now if you don't take this seriously." The outcome of the meeting was that the Police Officer advised Michelle and Krista of the seriousness of the matter and recommended that the behavior stop immediately.

On March 9th, several days after this meeting, the officer explained that I did not have the ability to press charges due to the lack of physical evidence; however he asked that I continue to report all future incidents.

I was warned by Angela Phillips to keep everything confidential about the police matter. Angela said she had begun to receive phone calls about the incident and rumors were spreading. She insinuated that I would be blamed for any additional gossip going forward.

The behavior continued.

This time Glenda finally decided to come up with a plan, which she assured me would solve this whole problem.

Her plan was that I was no longer allowed to use the front door, which is the main entrance and also handicap accessible. I was, from now on, to use the back door when coming or going. The other girls would be allowed to use the front. Due to only having one hand it was difficult for me to open the back door without disability supports, but I complied without further argument.

I used the back door, even though it was a struggle for me, especially when carrying my lunch or purse, and other belongings, while the other girls were able to use the main door—the door with the disability supports, which neither of the girls required.

The back door had significantly less traffic, which provided no protection. I felt uncomfortable and unsafe while using this entrance.

I felt like I was being punished. I couldn't understand why this was happening to me. The terrible feeling in the pit of my stomach was something so unbearable that I can't even describe it with words, but I will try: it was the most awful, dreadful feeling ever. The stress of having to walk into a toxic workplace every morning to report for my shift was almost unbearable. After each shift, I worked an extra fifteen minutes, to avoid running into Michelle and Krista—as well as Sarah Brown and Antonella Alfarano, who also participated in bullying on the Sunday of the original incident in 2011.

* * *

A particularly terrifying incident occurred. As I was finishing my shift late one night, a man I had never seen before chased me out of the Pioneer Manor parking lot. He cut me off in the parking lot and I had to slam on my brakes; then he proceeded to follow me. I drove towards the valley and when we got to the top of McCrae Heights, he was right behind me with high beams on.

I was afraid to go home, so I didn't.

I drove around the valley for over an hour and he continued to follow me. It was right around midnight. Finally, I pulled into Cortina Pizza, and ran inside, begging the employees to call 911.

The man stayed outside and in his vehicle, presumably waiting for me to leave so he could continue the intimidation—but then the police arrived. Two Police Officers were on scene. Both of the officers spoke to him and then allowed him to leave, and then they spoke to me. I told the officer that I wanted him charged. The officer brushed me off, saying that the man had stated he had only followed me because he had suspected me of drunk driving—a story that did not even make sense because I had come out of Pioneer Manor in uniform, where there is no access to alcohol, and I got into a minivan to drive home. I definitely was not drunk. I truly believe this was set up by someone at Pioneer Manor. I know this because I have had no issues with anyone other than the employees at Pioneer Manor.

The Police Officers that night broke protocol. They both spoke to him first and then let him go before discussing with me. When I brought this up, they justified it as having been right to let him go because they believed his story.

I explained to the officers that this implied that I was free to do this to someone else—follow them around for an hour, high beams on—and it wouldn't be against the law. One of the officers interjected right away and said, "You can't do that, it's illegal".

"But you basically just told me it isn't," I argued.

I had never seen this guy before in my life, but he told the Police Officers that he lived in Capreol. I found that really hard to believe—had he lived in Capreol, I would have definitely seen him before. He had a fancy car and a license plate that started with 9F. That is all I could remember.

I insisted again that I wanted him charged, and they told me once more that it was not possible, so I gave up and went home.

I got the impression that the two Police Officers made an error that night when they released him without pressing charges. I felt they were aware of their mistake and they just wanted to sweep it under the rug. They wanted it to go away.

I pressed on with the matter. Later that night, with my child in the vehicle, I drove to a pay phone and called the chief of police. All he did was suggest that it was an ex-boyfriend. Again, I felt defeated and disheartened, like no one was listening to me.

Meanwhile, the appalling harassment at work continued on.

Michelle stood behind me in line at one point and loudly said, "You're never going to get away with this you stupid bitch" in front of other employees.

Out of almost five hundred employees, everyone at work stopped talking to me because they didn't want to get involved. They made a point to purposely avoid me, and to stay far away, for fear of having this happen to them. No one wanted to endure this same harassment and bullying by Michelle and Krista. I truly believe I wasn't the first and would not be the last to go through this at their hands.

Another intimidating incident had Michelle and Krista standing in the area where I was working, while on their break, even though they had no reason to be there. They stood there and laughed at me for over twenty minutes, and I reported it to Angela Phillips. Her response to me was "isn't break only fifteen minutes?"

"Exactly," I answered.

Angela still did nothing.

During one of our several meetings, Angela told me that she and Glenda Gauthier are friends, and I believe that to be why Angela had to stand behind Glenda's actions, whether she agreed with her or not.

* * *

On March 14, 2012, following a meeting involving Management, Krista, and Michelle, I was brought to the Emergency Department at Health Sciences North by my Disability Manager, Kristina Fink, and Union Representative, Julie Bisaillon. I had become distraught during the meeting when Krista jumped out of her seat and I believed she was going to physically attack me. Julie was concerned about my mental health and well-being. I agreed to remain hospitalized until the end of March.

I was discharged from the hospital on March 26, 2012, and prescribed various medications to help cope with the stress and anxiety stemming from the harassment and bullying I endured in the workplace.

The doctor stated that in his opinion, I would be better off working in another place at the City, rather than working at Pioneer Manor, for my own health and well-being.

I received a psychological report that stated that my emotional difficulties, depression and anxiety were a consequence of the workplace harassment, and my earlier concussion—no other stressors were identified. My depression was a direct result of being bullied by Michelle, Krista, and the other employees who took part.

I filed a WSIB claim for traumatic mental stress due to ongoing harassment and bullying and Christina Fink was assigned as my disability manager.

In October of 2012, the WSIB claim I submitted was denied because, although I was being bullied, the situation was not considered *life-threatening*, even though I had planned to end my life. The letter read: "The events are unfortunate, but I have not identified a life-threatening situation. I concluded that there are interpersonal issues between you and your co-workers. The situation does not meet the criteria of trauma as defined in the traumatic mental stress policy […]."

I continued to fall deeper into debt, due to my growing absences at work— unable to cope with the unnecessary stress of the environment, and having to stay home more and more often.

On December 21, 2012, Krista and Michelle walked by the front desk where I was sitting alone and they stood for several minutes, to intimidate me. I reported it to Angela and Glenda. They informed me that since there was no proof of this, they could not stop the behavior.

Fran Bonony, a union representative, attended a meeting with me on January 20, 2013, with Management, Krista and Michelle. Krista and Michelle became so verbally abusive that I began to cry, and ultimately had to leave the room. In an affidavit statement written by Fran Bonony, due to severe bullying, the meeting should have been stopped but Management did nothing to defuse the situation. The affidavit also states that Fran Bonony felt I was in a volatile situation in the meeting and the Supervisors failed to address the bullying, and that I shouldn't have had to face the two bullies without Management intervening.

On January 30, 2013, Krista Saille stood alone in the nursing station, just staring at me without saying anything. This intimidation was reported to Bony Cummings, Registered Nurse Supervisor, who reported it back to Management, but she took no further action—and again, nor did Management.

On February 14, 2013, I received an affidavit letter from Maria Mastroianni, Union Representative, regarding the meeting that was held on March 14, 2012. The letter stated that I was extremely emotional and I voiced my opinions on what I believed was harassment and bullying. I explained that I had been unable to cope due to the stress of the workplace. During the meeting, voices were raised and some coworkers got up and left. Due to the inability to resolve the issues, the meeting was adjourned. Again, I mentioned the inability to cope, as well as thoughts of suicide, and emotional distress—and still, no satisfactory solution was provided.

On May 30, 2013, I was in the staff room, picking up my pay stub. Michelle O'Connell walked in, stood directly behind me, and proceeded to laugh—even though she was not talking to anyone. I completely froze with fear. I stood there, frozen, like I wasn't even in my own body. I could hear her speak my name, but I couldn't do anything. I reported this to Amanda Godin, the Registered Nurse Program Coordinator, who simply apologized and explained that she'd stop the bullying if she could but she didn't know how.

* * *

Due to seniority and staff rotation, in June 2013 I was offered a full-time position by Pioneer Manor, in the Trillium area where Phalyn Sproule, and her mother Beverly worked.

I believe Beverly Sproule was always trying to get information out of me. She would say dramatic things such as, "you've got Pioneer Manor by the balls" and laugh.

This morning was no different, she attempted to grill me for information—but up until then Beverly had never actually been cruel to me.

An incident with Beverly occurred while she and I were with a resident that I was assisting in the dining area. Beverly grabbed a spoon out of my hand and smashed it down onto the plate of food, which splashed me in the face. Then she walked away.

Although I was upset, I assumed it was a one off event, and I thought nothing else of it.

After I accepted a full time position in her unit, I was assisting Beverly's daughter, Phalyn, in another area with an Alzheimer's resident who required two staff assistance. Phalyn was to watch the residents hands while I provided care but she decided to leave one hand free so she could text on her phone, restraining the resident with only one hand. The resident wriggled free and struck Phalyn in the face. Phalyn reacted by striking the resident back three times in the face. I stared at her, jaw-dropped and in shock. She pointed her finger at my face and said "if you say anything about this, you're next".

Fearing that I was going to come forward, Phalyn got to Management before I did and in an attempt to tarnish my reputation further, she and her mother convinced them that I had been going around saying "I have Pioneer Manor by the balls," when in fact she had been the one saying that all along.

I never brought this incident forward to management as I feared for my well-being.

Following this incident, I was told to take on a significantly larger workload than the other employees in my area by Beverly Sproule; a co-worker, not a manager.

At this time, Angela was no longer allowed to speak with me and I was to bring any concerns to Judith Comtois if there were any work related issues going forward. I met with Judith and I explained that the workload I had been asked to take on was unfair, and was heavier than what the other girls were required to do. I had twelve residents to care for. Beverly Sproule only had six, and was just as capable as I was, and had the use of both her hands. It was extremely unreasonable. Judith told me to just do whatever Beverly ordered, even though Beverly was not a supervisor; she was just my co-worker. I objected.

"Just do what you're told," Judith had replied, rudely, and that was the end of that conversation.

* * *

On October 12, 2013, I received an upsetting and unprofessional Facebook message from Rick O'Connell, who was the Union President, and husband of Michelle O'Connell. He wrote "Hey. Seen your Facebook posting. I have a copy of it and

Glenda and Tony are going to see it Tuesday. I won't let this go. I'm going after your job. People like you are so unhappy in your own life that you feed off this. Remember this, if you harass someone outside of work it's the same as doing it at work. Everyone knows who you were talking about and it's the same as saying my name."

He was accusing me of writing something about his wife, Michelle, on Facebook, which was untrue—I made sure not to post work-related comments on Facebook, and I would have never written something so specific about a co-worker. The Facebook incident he was referring to was that Monique Grignon was running for president and I had sent her Facebook message saying "I hope you get it because you deserve it and you know your stuff". He took this message from Facebook and claimed that I was speaking poorly of him, and was hoping someone else would get the position.

I was not sure of how Rick O'Connell was able to see my Facebook in the first place. I didn't have him as a friend on Facebook, and I had cleaned up my friends list. At this time, I felt it best to clean up my friends list again—I removed everyone I couldn't trust, including Ina Horne, a Union Representative and Personal Support Worker I had once trusted but now realized probably did not have my best interest at heart. Right before I removed her from Facebook, I overheard

Tony Parmar tell her to keep an eye on me, and she agreed to.

This meant that there was one more person against me; someone who should have protected me.

I also had Annette on Facebook, who was a coworker in the same area as Rick. She falsely claimed to be a friend of mine. She never personally did anything to me so I had no reason to believe otherwise, however I found out afterwards that she was the one who had gone through my Facebook and randomly picked out stuff to show Rick, claiming I'd posted about Michelle.

I had trusted Ina, despite having heard that when I started, she and Julie Bisaillon had said that by hiring me, Pioneer

Manor 'went all to Hell', that I would never last, and that they would be sure not to help me. I believe in my heart now that they did indeed say these things.

Eventually I felt it best to get away from social media, and I deleted my entire Facebook account.

Pioneer Manor added the written warning to my file, stating that I had probably said something on Facebook. I was disciplined for a probability. I fought it. I voiced my concerns in a meeting with Tony Parmar, Glenda Gauthier and Fran Bonony, and explained that it was not fair, and finally I was told it would not go on my file. I found out afterwards that it had.

Right after this, I was informed that during an investigation, Pioneer Manor had decided that the message from Rick was inappropriate and that he would be reprimanded, although I never found out what the outcome of that discipline was, and things remained normal.

* * *

I continued to miss more work. I walked out of a meeting because I had anxiety and couldn't face this any longer. As outlined in the lawsuit, the bullying was playing so much on my emotions that I was experiencing a great deal of stress and anxiety, causing me to have to miss work. I had to miss so many shifts because I felt it was not a safe workplace that my bills began to pile up and I ended up seriously behind. I received notices from my mortgage company and disconnection notices from my utility companies.

In 2014, both my vehicle and my house were repossessed, and I was forced to move into a one bedroom apartment, where I slept on a reclining chair so that my child could have the bedroom.

* * *

I couldn't take anymore of the daily harassment or the things I had witnessed over two years, in combination with the fact that I had sustained a head injury at work, I went on a medical leave, with the understanding that I would return when the toxic environment had been made safe for me to work in. Angela Phillips took me aside and told me everything was in my head. I was never able to return to work at Pioneer Manor. In October of 2014 I received my vacation pay out, so I contacted Unemployment to find out why I had been paid out. They explained that I had been terminated for misconduct and claimed that they had sent a letter to me by mail in September. The letter was not a registered letter, and I had never received it. When I inquired about my employee file, Pioneer Manor had two different dates that I had apparently been terminated on, and they were never clear as to when this had supposedly happened or why.

I fought the dismissal. I spoke with several different people. I pushed forward with my lawsuit. I fought this as hard as I could.

I became even more severely depressed and suicidal.

* * *

Pioneer Manor took everything from me.

To this day, I still have no income other than a disability check.

I used to have a 4 bedroom house with a pool, and a vehicle, but I couldn't keep up with any of the payments and I lost it all. Pioneer Manor put me into $35,000 worth of debt by letting me go, after I witnessed things that no personal support worker working in a long-term care facility should have to witness; things that I should have never had to endure myself. After years of harassment and being bullied. Years of discrimination. Years of no one listening to me.

I raised my son by myself and worked hard for everything I had, and then I lost it all because I could no longer work in a toxic environment, with people who were hungover and drunk almost daily, who would not pull their weight, and who physically abused residents. I was called names, cursed at and laughed at, simply because I had gone in to help and the other employees were too drunk, too hungover, or just too lazy to do their share of the work.

During my employment at Pioneer Manor, I had witnessed two employees, Sarah Brown, who is a nurse and supervisor, and Krista Saile, doing cocaine at a bar where I was with another co-worker named Cindy, who had asked me to be her designated driver. Cindy would never confirm this, for fear of getting involved and becoming the next victim.

* * *

In 2014, I decided to pursue legal action, and Pioneer Manor was officially served by my legal team for events that took place up until October 17, 2014. The lawsuit named Krista Saile, Michelle O'Connell, Glenda Gauthier (Manager),

Tony Parmar (Director) and Pioneer Manor as a whole as respondents.

The lawsuit spoke of the original incident on March 13, 2011; about how I was called in to work in The Lodge, where Krista and Michelle had me do double the amount of work I should have, and still accused me of doing nothing all morning, and where they told me I would be responsible for caring for the last three residents by myself and I would receive no help at all.

It spoke of my work injury, and other incidents, including May 23, 2011, when I was walking into Pioneer Manor, and Michelle and Krista approached me and said "you better keep your mouth shut and not say anything", and various other incidents.

It spoke of how they both followed me around, just to stand and laugh or stare for periods of time, to intimidate me.

It spoke of how I had been constantly threatened and I was afraid for my safety.

Up until this point I had a clean employee record, other than the Facebook incident and my absences. I was an exceptional employee with acceptable attendance. There was nothing on my file—until Pioneer Manor was served by my legal team.

Then, there were lies, and more lies.

Suddenly in 2014 there were things on my file that had not been there before.

Someone at Pioneer Manor was making things up to hurt my credibility, trying to make it impossible for me to pursue legal action.

* * *

All of this happened to me because I had gone in on a Sunday; on my day off—a shift I was not originally scheduled to work—a shift I went in for because I was a good person and a dedicated employee, and I put my whole heart into my career.

I didn't have to go in on that Sunday, and I certainly wouldn't have had I known I was about to get bullied for the next two years of my life.

Sarah Brown Brown eventually apologized for bullying me, and she was never named in my court documents, nor was Antonella Alfarano, because she had only joined in with the other girls to prevent also becoming a victim of the harassment.

Michelle O'Connell and Sarah Brown were eventually terminated from Pioneer Manor.

Krista Saile, Antonella Alfarano, Phalyn Sproule, and Beverly Sproule, still work at Pioneer Manor, as of right now. As far as I am aware, Glenda Gauthier (Nursing Manager), Angela Phillips (Program Coordinator) and Tony Parmar (Director), are also still working at Pioneer Manor. Horrifying things happen there to people's loved ones, and everyone turns a blind eye. The behavior of the employees, the drug abuse, and the treatment of the residents at Pioneer Manor is unacceptable and needs to be made public.

I will not rest until the truth is known and big changes are made. I cannot sleep comfortably at night, knowing that no one else will stand up for the residents of Pioneer Manor.

ABOUT THE AUTHOR

Tammy Rector is a disabled, single mother who resides in Greater Sudbury. She desperately hopes that this truthful account of events that took place in her workplace will shed some light on the things that go on in Pioneer Manor, a Long-Term Care facility run by the City of Greater Sudbury.